The Complete Pescatarian Cookbook

Dozens Tasty and easy-to-prepare
Recipes for the whole family

Lara Dillard

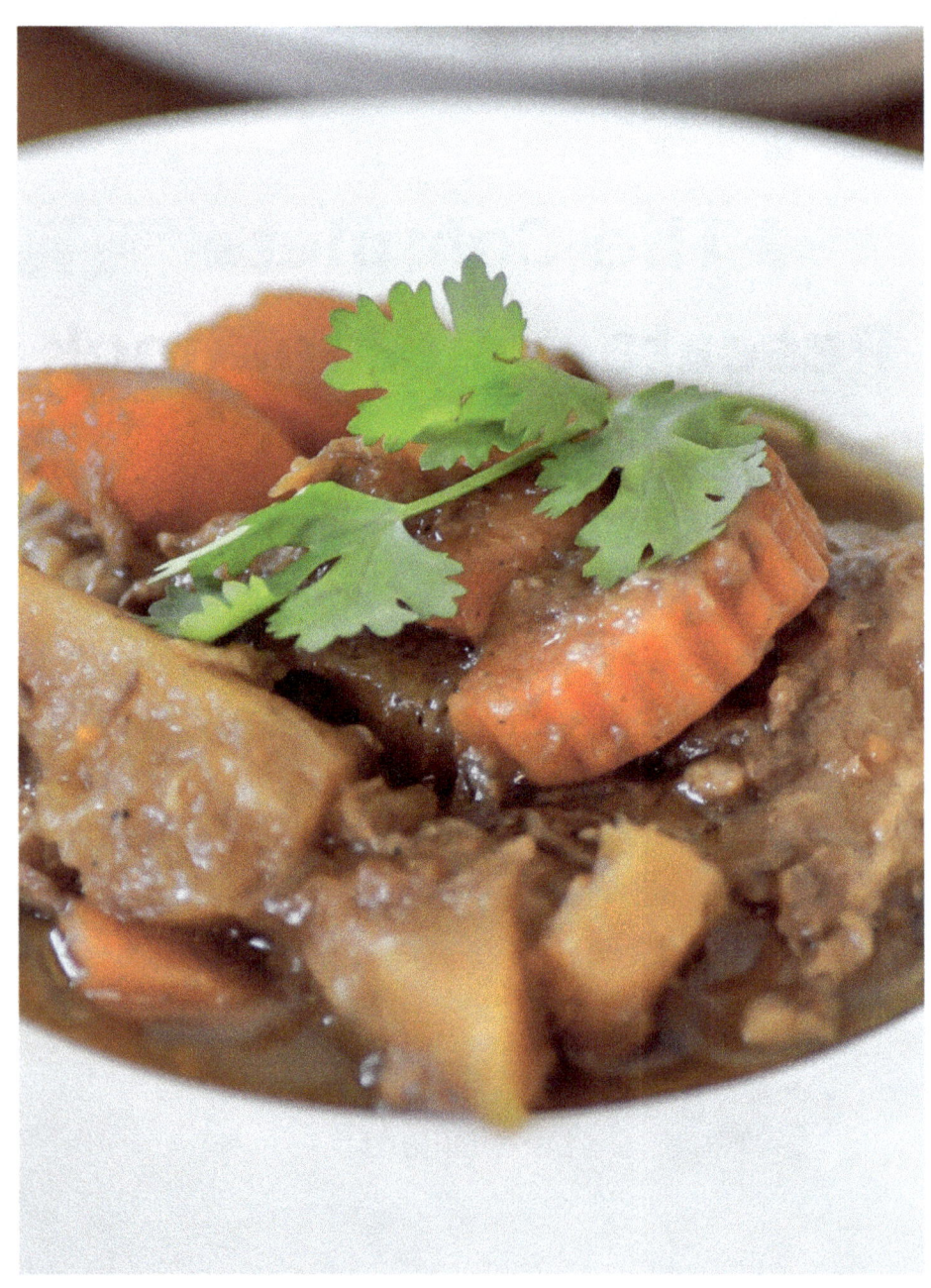

© copyright 2021 – all rights reserved.

the content contained within this book may not be reproduced, duplicated or transmitted without direct written permission from the author or the publisher.

under no circumstances will any blame or legal responsibility be held against the publisher, or author, for any damages, reparation, or monetary loss due to the information contained within this book. either directly or indirectly.

legal notice:

this book is copyright protected. this book is only for personal use. you cannot amend, distribute, sell, use, quote or paraphrase any part, or the content within this book, without the consent of the author or publisher.

disclaimer notice:

please note the information contained within this document is for educational and entertainment purposes only. all effort has been executed to present accurate, up to date, and reliable, complete information. no warranties of any kind are declared or implied. readers acknowledge that the author is not engaging in the rendering of legal, financial, medical or professional advice. the content within this book has been derived from various sources. please consult a licensed professional before attempting

any techniques outlined in this book.

by reading this document, the reader agrees that under no circumstances is the author responsible for any losses, direct or indirect, which are incurred as a result of the use of information contained within this document, including, but not limited to, — errors, omissions, or inaccuracies.

Table of Contents

Monastery Stew	6
Rice with Spinach	8
Eggplant and Chickpea Stew	10
Turkish Green Beans	12
Rice and Cabbage Stew	14
Roasted Red Pepper Soup	17
Vegetarian Gazpacho	19
Creamy Zucchini Soup	21
Celery Root Soup	23
Moroccan Lentil Soup	25
Delicious Minestrone Soup	27
Beet and Carrot Soup	29
Green Lentil Soup with Rice	32
Broccoli and Potato Soup	34
Tomato Soup with Rice	36
Chickpea and Carrot Soup	38
Spiced Carrot Soup	40
Mushroom, Barley and Lentil Soup	42
Creamy Wild Mushroom Soup	44
Mediterranean Buckwheat Salad	46
Beet and Bean Sprout Salad	48
Tasty Tabbouleh	50
Savory Fatoush	52
Chickpea Salad	55
Red Cabbage Salad	57
Zucchini Salad with Greek Yogurt	59
Cucumber Salad	61

Carrot Salad with Yogurt	64
Strained Yogurt Salad	66
Turkish Beet Salad with Yogurt	68
Spinach Stem Salad	70
Roasted Eggplant and Pepper Relish	73
Kale Salad with Creamy Tahini Dressing	75
Brown Lentil Salad	77
Bulgur with Walnuts and Green Lentils	79
Slimming Ginger Steamed Fish	81
One Pan Baked Teriyaki Salmon	83
Blackened Fish Tacos with Cabbage Mango Slaw	86
Garlic Lemon Scallops	89
Shrimp & Broccoli in Chili Sauce	92
Prawn Pitta Scoops	94
Shrimp with Cilantro and Lime	96
Maple Mustard Salmon	98
Grilled Shrimp Marinade with Shrimp Sauce	99
Mexi' Shrimp Salad Wrap	101
Fish and Shrimp Stew	103

Monastery Stew

Servings: 4

Ingredients and Quantity

- 3 to 4 potatoes, diced
- 2 to 3 tomatoes, diced
- 1 to 2 carrots, chopped
- 1 to 2 onions, finely chopped
- 1 cup small shallots, whole
- 1 celery rib, chopped
- 2 cups fresh mushrooms, chopped
- 1/2 cup black olives, pitted
- 1/4 cup rice
- 1/2 cup white wine
- 1/2 cup sunflower oil
- 1 bunch parsley
- 1 tsp. black pepper
- 1 tsp. salt

Direction

1. Sauté the finely chopped onions, carrots and celery in a little oil.
2. Add the small onions, olives, mushrooms and black pepper and then stir well.
3. Pour over the wine and 1 cup of water, salt to your taste.
4. Cover and allow to simmer until tender.
5. After 15 minutes, add the diced potatoes, the rice and the tomato pieces.
6. Transfer everything into a clay pot, sprinkle with parsley and bake for about 30 minutes at 350 degrees F. Serve and enjoy!

Rice with Spinach

Servings: 4

Ingredients and Quantity

- 3 to 4 cups fresh spinach, washed, drained and chopped
- 1/2 cup rice
- 1 onion, chopped
- 1 carrot, chopped
- 1/4 cup extra virgin olive oil
- 2 cups water

Direction

1. Heat the oil in a large skillet and cook the onions and the carrots until soft.
2. Add the paprika and the washed, rinsed and drained rice and then mix well.

3. Add 2 cups of warm water, stirring constantly as the rice absorbs it.
4. Simmer for more 20 minutes.
5. Wash the spinach well and cut in strips.
6. Add the rice and cook until it wilts.
7. Remove from the heat and season to taste. Serve with yogurt. Enjoy!

Eggplant and Chickpea Stew

Servings: 4

Ingredients and Quantity

- 2 to 3 eggplants, peeled and diced
- 1 onion, chopped
- 2 to 3 garlic cloves, crushed
- 1 can (15 oz.) chickpeas, drained
- 1 can (15 oz.) tomatoes, undrained, diced
- 1 tsp. paprika
- 1/2 tsp. cinnamon
- 1 tsp. cumin
- 1 tbsp. olive oil
- Salt and pepper, to taste

Direction

1. Peel and dice the eggplants.

2. Heat olive oil in a large deep frying pan and sauté onions and crushed garlic.
3. Add paprika, cumin and cinnamon. Stir well to coat evenly.
4. Sauté for 3 to 4 minutes until the onions are soft.
5. Add the eggplant, tomatoes and chickpeas.
6. Bring to a boil, lower the heat and simmer for 10 minutes, covered or until the eggplant is tender.
7. Uncover the simmer for a few more minutes until the liquid evaporates. Serve and enjoy!

Turkish Green Beans

Servings: 4

Ingredients and Quantity

- 1 lb. green beans, fresh or frozen
- 1 onion, chopped
- 4 garlic cloves, crushed
- 2 large tomatoes, diced
- 1/4 cup sunflower oil
- 1/2 cup hot water
- 1 tbsp. paprika
- 1/4 tsp. cumin
- 1 tsp. salt
- 1 tsp. sugar
- Black pepper, to taste
- 1 bunch fresh parsley, chopped, for serving

Direction

1. Sauté the onions and the garlic lightly in olive oil.
2. Add the green beans and the remaining ingredients.
3. Cover and simmer over medium heat for about an hour or until all vegetables are tender.
4. Check after 30 minutes; add more water if necessary.
5. Sprinkle with fresh parsley. Best served warm. Enjoy!

Rice and Cabbage Stew

Servings: 4

Ingredients and Quantity

- 1 cup long grain white rice
- 2 cups water
- 2 tbsp. extra virgin olive oil
- 1 small onion, chopped
- 1 garlic clove, crushed
- 1/4 head cabbage, cored and shredded
- 2 tomatoes, diced
- 1 tbsp. paprika
- 1/2 bunch parsley
- Salt, to taste
- Black pepper, to taste

Direction

1. Heat the olive oil in a large pot.

2. Add the onion and f=garlic and cook until transparent.
3. Add the paprika, rice and water and then stir and bring to a boil.
4. Simmer for 10 minutes.
5. Add the shredded cabbage, the tomatoes, and cook for about 20 minutes, stirring occasionally until the cabbage cooks down.
6. Season with salt and pepper.
7. Sprinkle with parsley. Serve and enjoy!

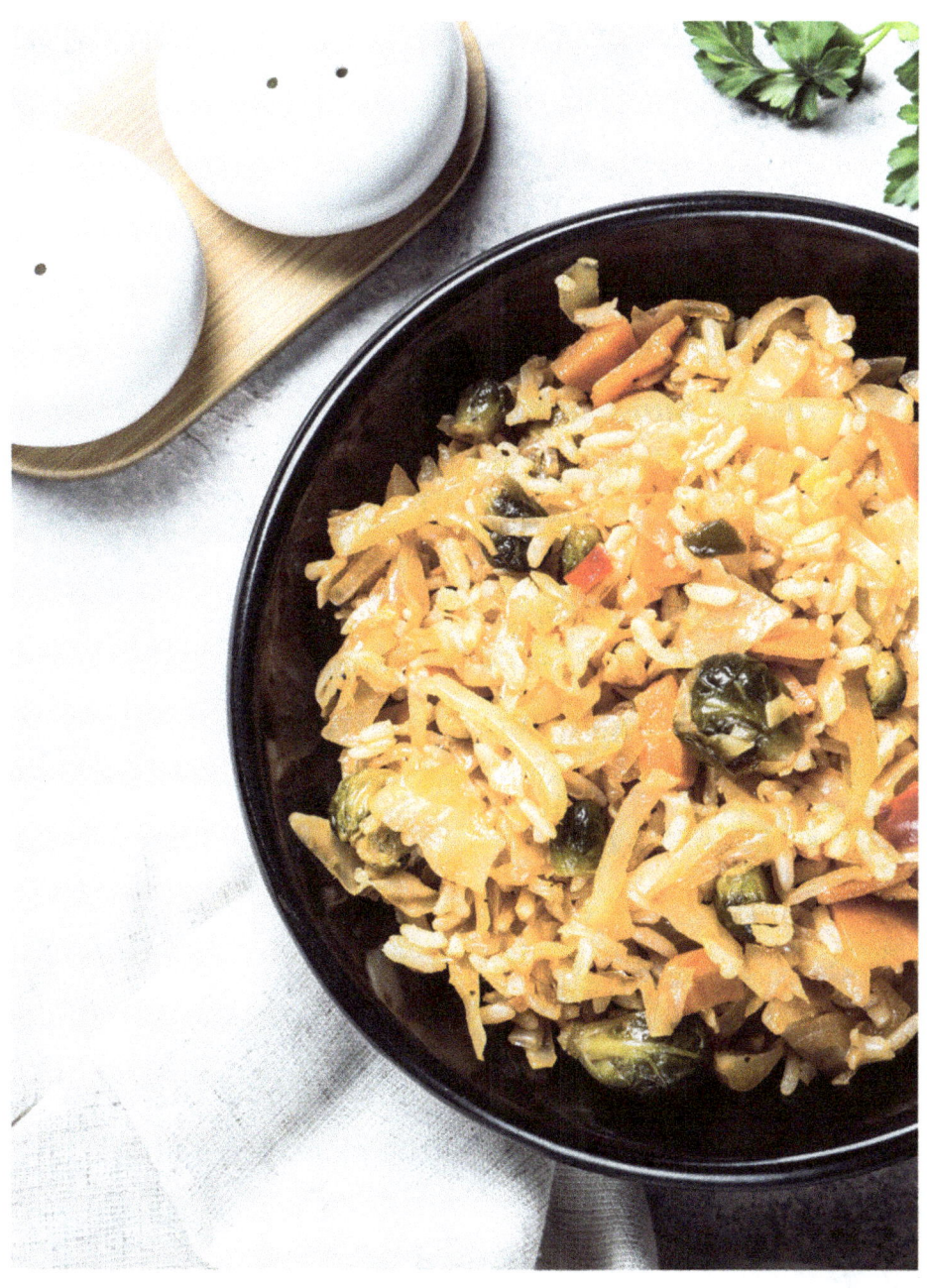

Roasted Red Pepper Soup

Servings: 6

Ingredients and Quantity

- 5 red peppers or more
- 1 large brown onion, chopped
- 2 garlic cloves, crushed
- 4 medium tomatoes, chopped
- 2 cups vegetable broth
- 3 tbsp. olive oil
- 2 bay leaves

Direction

1. Grill the peppers or roast them in the oven at 400 degrees F until the skins are a little burnt.

2. Place the roasted peppers in a brown paper bag or a lidded container and leave covered for about 10 minutes.
3. This makes it easier to peel them.
4. Peel the skins and remove the seeds.
5. Cut the peppers in small pieces.
6. Heat oil in a large saucepan over medium-high heat.
7. Add onion and garlic and sauté, stirring, for 3 minutes, or until onion has softened.
8. Add the red peppers, bay leaves, tomatoes and simmer for about 5 minutes.
9. Add broth and season with pepper.
10. Bring to boil and then reduce heat and simmer for 20 more minutes.
11. Set aside to cool slightly.
12. Blend in batches, until smooth. Serve and enjoy!

Vegetarian Gazpacho

Servings: 6

Ingredients and Quantity

- 2 1/4 lb. tomatoes, peeled and halved
- 1 onion, sliced
- 1 green pepper, sliced
- 1 big cucumber, peeled and diced
- 2 garlic cloves
- Salt, to taste
- 4 tbsp. olive oil
- 1 tbsp. apple vinegar

For Garnishing:

- 1/2 onion, chopped
- 1 green pepper, chopped
- 1 cucumber, chopped

Direction

1. Place the tomatoes, garlic, onion, green pepper, cucumber, salt, olive oil and vinegar in a blender or food processor and puree until smooth.

2. Add small amount of cold water if necessary to achieve desired consistency.

3. Serve the gazpacho chilled with the chopped onion, green pepper and cucumber. Enjoy!

Creamy Zucchini Soup

Servings: 4

Ingredients and Quantity

- 1 onion, finely chopped
- 2 garlic cloves, crushed
- 1 cup vegetable broth
- 2 cups water
- 2 zucchinis, peeled, thinly sliced
- 1 big potato, peeled and chopped
- 3 tbsp. olive oil
- 1/4 cup fresh basil leaves
- 1/2 cup yogurt, for serving

Direction

1. Heat olive oil in a saucepan over a medium heat.

2. Gently sauté onion and garlic for 1 to 2 minutes.
3. Add in vegetable broth and water and then bring to a boil.
4. Add in the zucchinis, potato and a teaspoon of sugar.
5. Reduce heat to medium-low and simmer, stirring occasionally, for 10 minutes or until the zucchinis are soft.
6. Stir in basil and simmer for 2-3 minutes more.
7. Set aside to cool, then blend in batches and reheat.
8. Serve with a dollop of yogurt and/or sprinkled with Parmesan cheese. Enjoy!

Celery Root Soup

Servings: 4

Ingredients and Quantity

- 2 leeks, the white and green parts only, chopped
- 2 garlic cloves, crushed
- 1 large celery root, peeled and diced
- 2 potatoes, peeled and diced
- 4 cups vegetable broth
- 1 bay leaf
- 2 tbsp. extra virgin olive oil
- Salt and black pepper, to taste

Direction

1. In a skillet, heat olive oil, then add the leeks and sauté about 3-4 minutes.
2. Add in the garlic and sauté an additional 3-40 seconds.

3. In a slow cooker, add the sautéed leeks and garlic, celeriac, potatoes, broth, bay leaf, salt, and pepper.
4. Cover and cook on low heat for 7-8 hours.
5. Set aside to cool.
6. Now, remove the bay leaf, then process in a blender or with an immersion blender until smooth. Serve and enjoy!

Moroccan Lentil Soup

Servings: 10

Ingredients and Quantity

- 1 cup red lentils
- 1 cup canned chickpeas, drained
- 2 onions, chopped
- 2 garlic cloves, minced
- 1 cup canned tomatoes, chopped
- 1 cup canned white beans, drained
- 3 carrots, diced
- 3 celery ribs, diced
- 4 cups water
- 3 tbsp. olive oil
- 1 tsp. ginger, grated
- 1 tsp. ground cardamom
- 1/2 tsp. ground cumin

Direction

1. In a large pot, sauté onions, garlic and ginger in olive oil for about 5 minutes.
2. Add the water, lentils, chickpeas, white beans, tomatoes, carrots, celery, cardamom and cumin.
3. Bring to a boil for a few minutes, then simmer for half an hour or longer until the lentils are tender.
4. Puree half the soup in a food processor or blender.
5. Return the pureed soup to the pot, stir and serve. Enjoy!

Delicious Minestrone Soup

Servings: 6

Ingredients and Quantity

- 1/4 cabbage, chopped
- 2 carrots, chopped
- 1 celery rib, thinly sliced
- 1 small onion, chopped
- 2 garlic cloves, chopped
- 2 cups water
- 1 cup canned tomatoes, diced, undrained
- 1 cup fresh spinach, torn
- 1/2 cup pasta, cooked

- 2 tbsp. extra virgin olive oil
- Black pepper and salt, to taste

Direction

1. Sauté the carrots, cabbage, celery, onion and garlic in oil for 5 minutes in a deep saucepan.
2. Add water, tomatoes and bring to a boil.
4. Reduce heat and simmer uncovered, for 20 minutes or until vegetables are tender.
5. Stir in spinach, macaroni, and season with salt and pepper to your taste. Serve and enjoy!

Beet and Carrot Soup

Servings: 6

Ingredients and Quantity

- 4 beets, washed and peeled
- 2 carrots, peeled, chopped
- 2 potatoes, peeled, chopped
- 1 medium sized onion, chopped
- 2 cups vegetable broth
- 2 cups water
- 2 tbsp. yogurt
- 2 tbsp. olive oil
- 1 bunch of spring onions, cut, for serving

Direction

1. Peel and chop the beets.

2. Heat olive oil in a saucepan over medium high heat and sauté onion and carrot until onion is tender.
3. Add beets, potatoes, broth and water.
4. Bring to the boil.
5. Reduce heat to medium and simmer, partially covered, for 30-40 minutes, or until beets are tender. Cool slightly.
6. Blend soup in batches until smooth.
7. Return it to pan over low heat and cook, stirring, for 4 to 5 minutes.
8. Serve with soup topped with yogurt and sprinkled with spring onions. Enjoy!

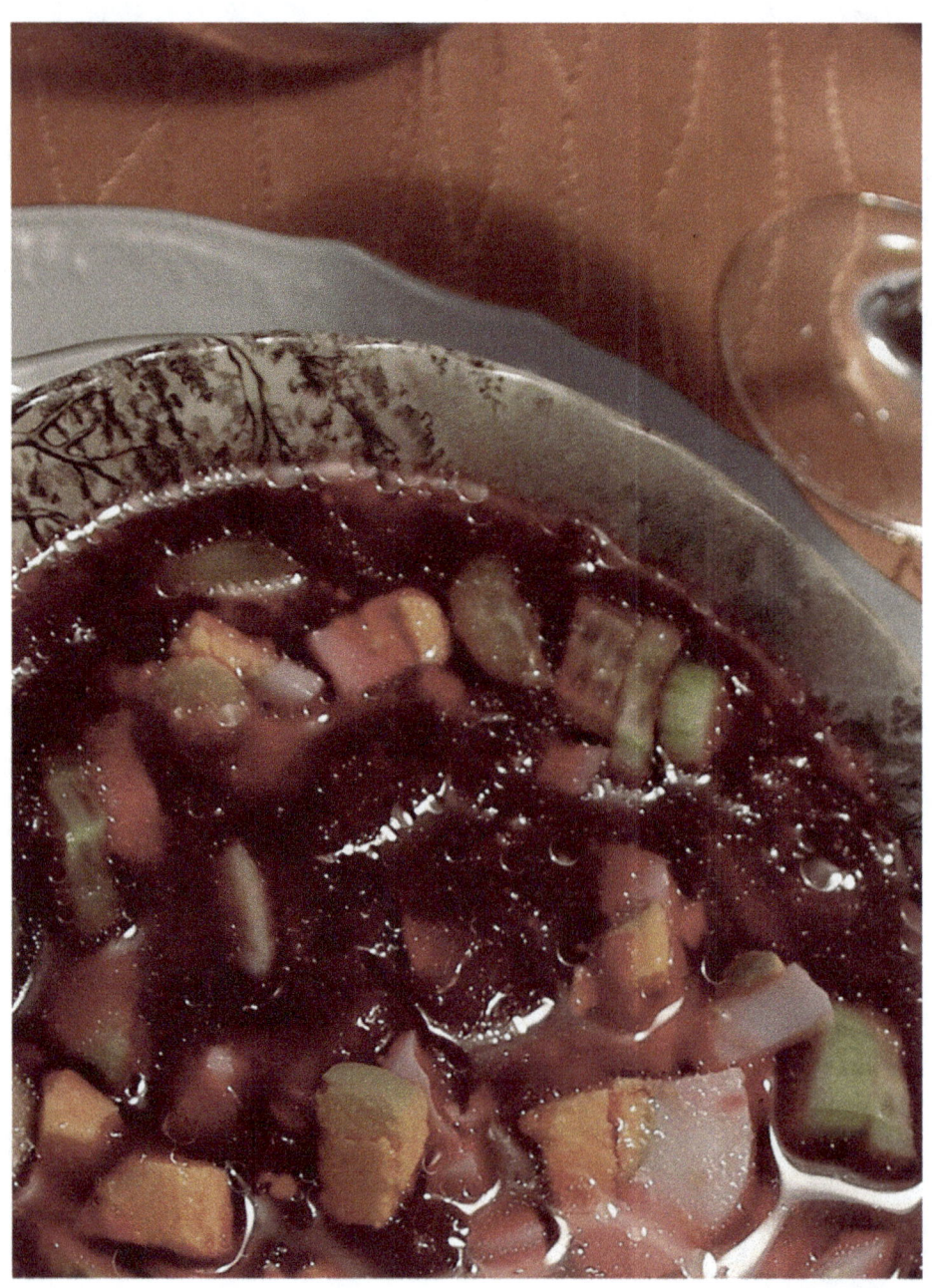

Green Lentil Soup with Rice

Servings: 6

Ingredients and Quantity

- 1 cup green lentils
- 1 small onion, finely cut
- 1 carrot, chopped
- 5 cups vegetable broth
- 1/4 cup rice
- 1 tbsp. paprika
- Salt and black pepper, to taste
- 1/2 cup finely cut dill, to serve

Direction

1. Heat oil in a large saucepan and sauté the onion stirring occasionally, until transparent.

2. Add in carrot, paprika and lentils and stir to combine.
3. Add vegetable broth to the saucepan and bring to the boil, then reduce heat and simmer for 20 minutes.
4. Stir in rice and cook on medium low until rice is properly cooked.
5. Sprinkle with dill. Serve and enjoy!

Broccoli and Potato Soup

Servings: 6

- **Ingredients and Quantity**
- 2 lb. broccoli, cut into florets
- 2 potatoes, chopped
- 1 big onion, chopped
- 3 garlic cloves, crushed
- 4 cups water
- 1 tbsp. olive oil
- 1/4 tsp. ground nutmeg

Direction

1. Heat oil in a large saucepan over medium-high heat.
2. Add onion and garlic and sauté, stirring, for 3 minutes, or until soft.
3. Add broccoli, potato and 4 cups of cold water.

5. Cover and bring to the boil, then reduce heat to low.
6. Simmer, stirring, for 10 to 15 minutes, or until the potatoes are tender.
7. Remove from heat and then blend until smooth.
8. Return to pan. Cook for 5 minutes or until properly cooked. Serve and enjoy!

Tomato Soup with Rice

Servings: 4

Ingredients and Quantity

- 1 large onion, diced
- 1/3 cup rice
- 3 cups water
- 2 garlic cloves, chopped
- 3 tbsp. olive oil
- 1/2 tsp. salt
- ½ tsp. black pepper
- 1 tsp. sugar
- ½ bunch fresh parsley

Direction

1. Sauté onion and garlic in oil in a large soup pot.
2. When onions have softened, add tomatoes and cook for 10 minutes.

3. Stir in the spices and sugar and mix well to coat vegetables.
4. Add water and simmer for 10 minutes and then stir in rice and cook for at least 20 minutes or till the rice is well cooked.
5. Sprinkle with parsley. Serve and enjoy!

Chickpea and Carrot Soup

Servings: 4

Ingredients and Quantity

- 4 big carrots, chopped
- 1 leek, chopped
- 4 cups vegetable broth
- 1 cup canned chickpeas, undrained
- 1/2 cup orange juice
- 2 tbsp. olive oil
- 1/2 tsp. cumin
- 1/2 tsp. ginger
- tbsp. yogurt, for serving

Direction

1. Heat oil in a large saucepan over medium heat.
2. Add leek and carrots and sauté until soft.

3. Add orange juice, broth, chickpeas and spices.
4. Bring to the boil.
5. Reduce heat to medium-low and simmer, covered, for 15 minutes.
6. Blend soup until smooth; return to pan.
7. Season with salt and pepper. Stir over heat until heated through.
8. Pour in about 4 bowls.
9. Top with yogurt. Serve and enjoy!

Spiced Carrot Soup

Servings: 6

Ingredients and Quantity

- 10 carrots, peeled and chopped
- 2 medium sized onions, chopped
- 4 cups water or more
- 2 garlic cloves, minced
- 1 big red chili pepper, finely chopped
- 5 tbsp. olive oil
- 1/2 bunch, fresh coriander, finely cut
- Salt and pepper, to taste
- /2 cup heavy cream

Direction

1. Heat the olive oil in a large pot over medium heat and sauté the onions, carrots, garlic and chili pepper until tender.

2. Add 4-5 cups of water and bring to a boil.
3. Reduce heat to low and simmer for 30 minutes.
4. Transfer the soup to a blender or food processor and blend until smooth.
5. Return to the pot and continue cooking for a few more minutes.
6. Remove the soup from heat and stir in the cream.
7. Serve with coriander sprinkled over each serving. Enjoy!

Mushroom, Barley and Lentil Soup

Servings: 4

Ingredients and Quantity

- 2 medium leeks, trimmed, halved, sliced
- 10 white mushrooms, sliced
- 3 garlic cloves, cut
- 2 bay leaves
- 2 cans tomatoes, chopped, undrained
- 3/4 cup red lentils
- 1/3 cup barley
- 3 tbsp. extra virgin olive oil
- 1 tsp. paprika
- 1 tsp. savory
- 1/2 tsp. cumin

Direction

1. Heat oil in a large saucepan over medium-high heat.
2. Sauté leeks and mushrooms for 3 to 4 minutes or until softened.
3. Add cumin, paprika, savory and tomatoes, lentils, barley and 5 cups cold water.
4. Season with salt and pepper.
5. Cover and bring to a boil. Reduce the heat to low.
6. Simmer for 35 to 40 minutes or until barley is tender. Serve and enjoy!

Creamy Wild Mushroom Soup

Servings: 4

Ingredients and Quantity

- 2 cups wild mushrooms, peeled and chopped
- 1 onion, chopped
- 2 garlic cloves, crushed and chopped
- 1 tsp. dried thyme
- 3 cups vegetable broth
- Salt and pepper, to taste
- 3 tbsp. olive oil

Direction

1. Sauté onions and garlic in a large soup pot till transparent.
2. Add thyme and mushrooms.
3. Cook for 10 minutes then add the vegetable broth and simmer for another 10-20 minutes.
4. Blend, season and serve. Enjoy!

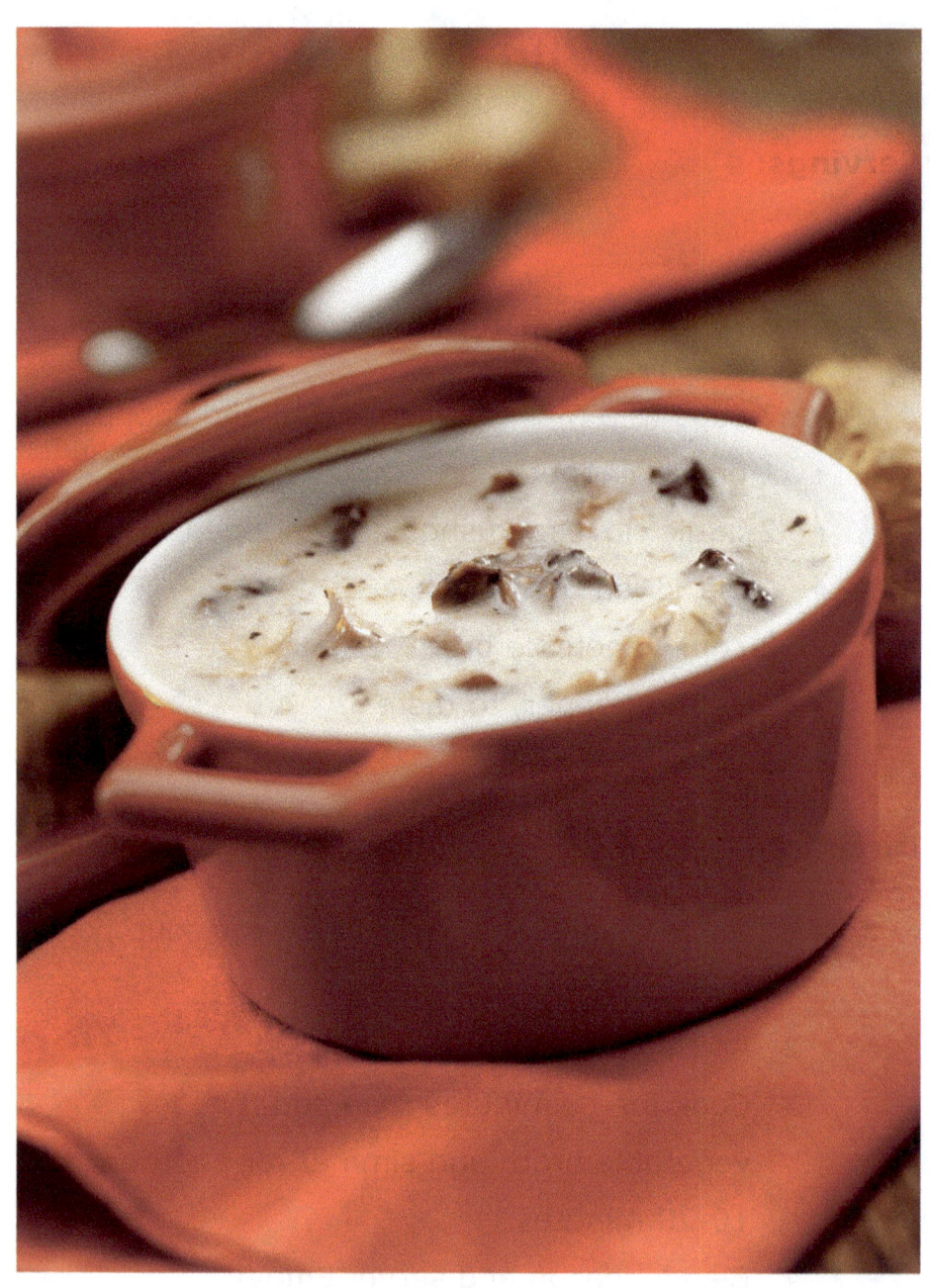

Mediterranean Buckwheat Salad

Servings: 4

Ingredients and Quantity

- 1 cup buckwheat grouts
- 1 3/4 cups water1 small red onion, finely chopped 1/2 cucumber, diced
- 1 cup cherry tomatoes, halved
- 1 yellow bell pepper, chopped
- A bunch parsley, finely cut
- 1 preserved lemon, finely chopped
- cup chickpeas, cooked or canned, drained Juice of half lemon
- 1 tsp. dried basil
- 2 tbsp. extra virgin olive oil
- Salt and black pepper, to taste

Direction

1. Heat a large, dry saucepan and toast the buckwheat for about 3 minutes.
2. Boil the water and add it carefully to the buckwheat.
3. Cover, reduce heat and simmer until buckwheat is tender and all liquid is absorbed (5-7 minutes).
4. Remove from heat, fluff with a fork and set aside to cool.
5. Mix the buckwheat with the chopped onion, bell pepper, cucumber, cherry tomatoes, parsley, preserved lemon and chickpeas in a salad bowl.
6. Whisk the lemon juice, olive oil and basil, season with salt and pepper to taste, then pour over the salad and stir.
7. Serve at room temperature. Enjoy!

Beet and Bean Sprout Salad

Servings: 4

Ingredients and Quantity

- 7 beet greens, finely sliced
- 2 medium tomatoes, sliced
- 1 cup bean sprouts, washed
- 2 garlic cloves, crushed
- 1/2 cup each for lemon juice, olive oil
- 1 tsp. salt

Direction

1. In a large bowl, toss together beet greens, bean sprouts, tomatoes, and dressing.
2. Mix oil and lemon juice with lemon rind, salt and garlic and pour over the salad.
3. Refrigerate for 2 hours to allow flavor to develop before serving.

4. Best served chilled. Enjoy!

Tasty Tabbouleh

Servings: 6

Ingredients and Quantity

- 1 cup raw bulgur
- 2 cups boiling water
- A bunch of parsley, finely cut
- 2 tomatoes, finely cut
- 2 tomatoes, chopped
- 3 tbsp. olive oil
- 2 garlic cloves, minced
- 6 to 7 fresh green onions, chopped
- 1 tbsp. fresh mint leaves, chopped
- Juice of 2 lemons
- Salt and black pepper, to taste

Direction

1. Bring water and salt to a boil, and then pour over bulgur.

2. Cover and set aside for 15 minutes to steam.
3. Drain excess water from bulgur and fluff with a fork. Leave it to chill.
4. In a large bowl, mix together the parsley, tomatoes, olive oil, garlic, green onions and mint.
5. Stir in the chilled bulgur and season to taste with salt, pepper and lemon juice. Serve and enjoy!

Savory Fatoush

Servings: 6

Ingredients and Quantity

- 2 cups lettuce, washed, dried and chopped
- 3 tomatoes, chopped
- 1 cucumber, peeled and chopped
- 1 green pepper, seeded and chopped
- 1/2 cup radishes, sliced in half
- 1 small red onion, finely chopped
- 1/2 bunch parsley, finely cut
- 2 tbsp. fresh mint, finely chopped
- 3 tbsp. extra virgin olive oil
- 4 tbsp. lemon juice
- Salt and black pepper, to taste
- 2 whole-wheat pita breads

Direction

1. Toast the pita breads in a skillet until they are browned and crispy. Then set aside.
2. Place the lettuce, tomatoes, cucumbers, green pepper, radishes, onion, parsley and mint in a salad bowl.
3. Break up the toasted pita into bite-size pieces and add to the salad.
4. Make the dressing by whisking together the olive oil with the lemon juice, a pinch of salt and some black pepper.
5. Toss everything together until vegetables are well coated with the dressing. Serve and enjoy!

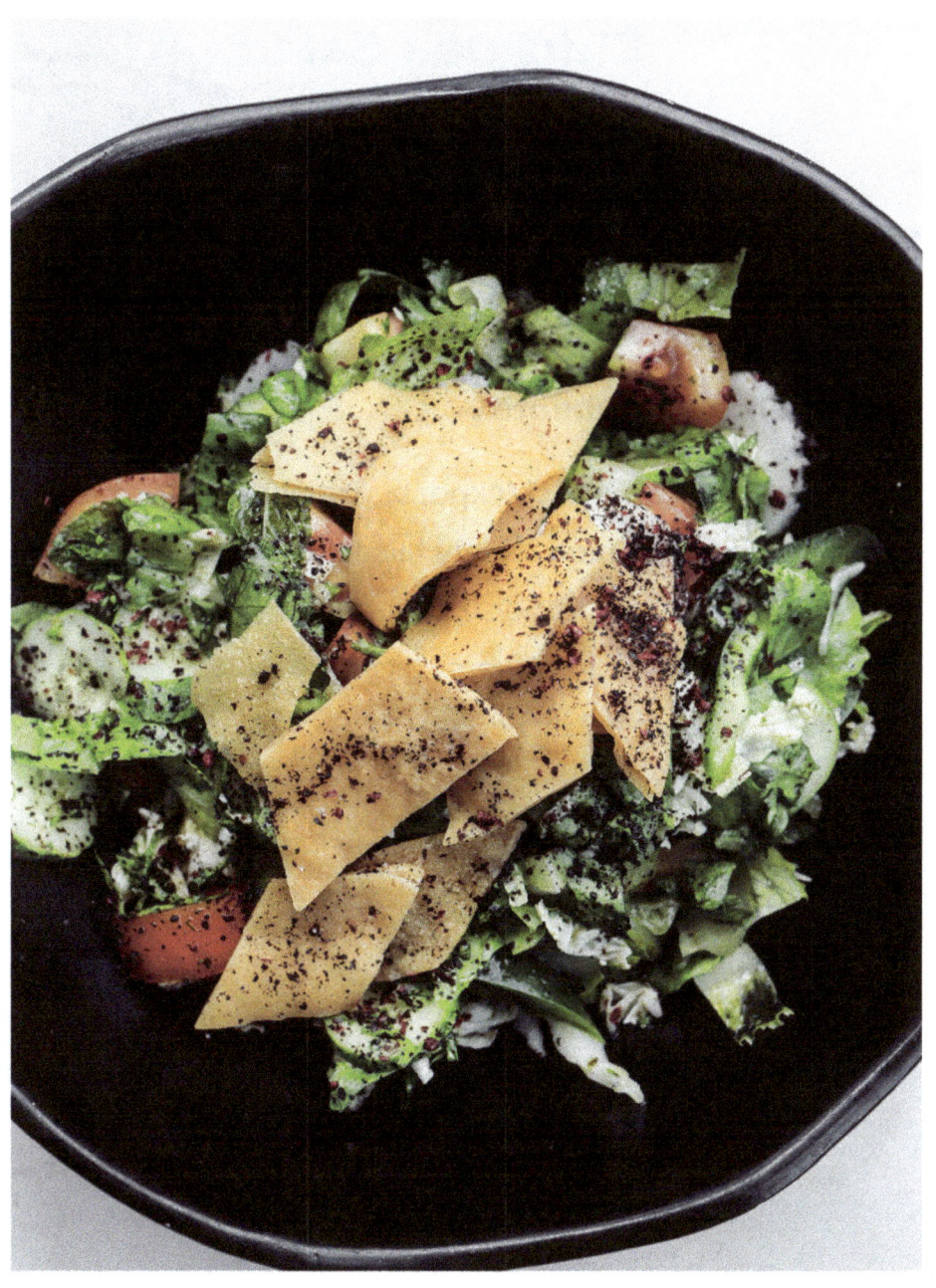

Chickpea Salad

Servings: 4

Ingredients and Quantity

- 1 cup canned chickpeas, drained and rinsed
- 1 spring onion, thinly sliced
- 1 small cucumber, deseeded and diced
- 2 green bell peppers, diced
- 2 tomatoes, diced
- 2 tsp. fresh parsley, chopped
- 1 tsp. capers, drained and rinsed
- Juice of 1/2 lemon
- 2 tbsp. extra virgin olive oil
- 1 tsp. balsamic vinegar
- Salt and pepper, to taste
- A pinch dried oregano

Direction

1. In a medium bowl, toss together the chickpeas, spring onion, cucumber, bell pepper, tomato, parsley, capers and lemon juice.
2. In a smaller bowl, stir together the remaining ingredients and pour over the chickpea salad.
3. Toss well to coat and allow to marinate, stirring occasionally, for at least one hour before serving. Enjoy!

Red Cabbage Salad

Servings: 6

Ingredients and Quantity

- 1 small head red cabbage, cored and chopped
- 1 bunch fresh dill, finely cut
- 3 tbsp. sunflower oil
- 3 tbsp. red wine vinegar
- 1 tsp. Sugar
- 2 tsp. salt
- Black pepper, to taste

Direction

1. In a cup, mix the sunflower oil, red wine vinegar, sugar and black pepper.
2. Place the cabbage in a large glass bowl.

3. Sprinkle the salt on top and crunch it with your hands to soften.
4. Pour dressing over the cabbage and toss to coat.

Sprinkle with dill, cover with foil and leave in the refrigerator for half an hour before serving. Enjoy!

Zucchini Salad with Greek Yogurt

Servings: 4

Ingredients and Quantity

- 3 medium zucchinis, coarsely chopped
- 1 cup Greek Yogurt
- 1/2 cup walnuts, crushed
- 2 garlic cloves, chopped
- 2 tbsp. extra virgin olive oil
- 1 tsp. paprika
- 1 tbsp. dried mint
- 1/2 cup fresh dill, finely cut
- Salt, to taste

Direction

1. Grate the zucchinis and squeeze them with your hands to drain excessive juice.
2. Heat the olive oil in a pan and gently cook zucchinis, stirring, for 4 to 5 minutes or until tender.
3. Stir in paprika and set aside to cool down.
4. When zucchinis have cooled down, add in garlic, walnuts, dill, mint and salt. Stir to combine well and add in yogurt.
5. Stir again. Best served cold. Enjoy!

Cucumber Salad

Servings: 4

Ingredients and Quantity

- 2 medium cucumbers, peeled and sliced
- A bunch fresh dill
- 2 to 3 cloves garlic, pressed
- 3 tbsp. white wine vinegar
- 3 tbsp. olive oil
- Salt, to taste

Direction

1. Cut the cucumbers in rings and put them in a salad bowl.
2. Add the finely cut dill, the pressed garlic and season with salt, vinegar and oil.

3. Toss to combine. Best served cold. Enjoy!

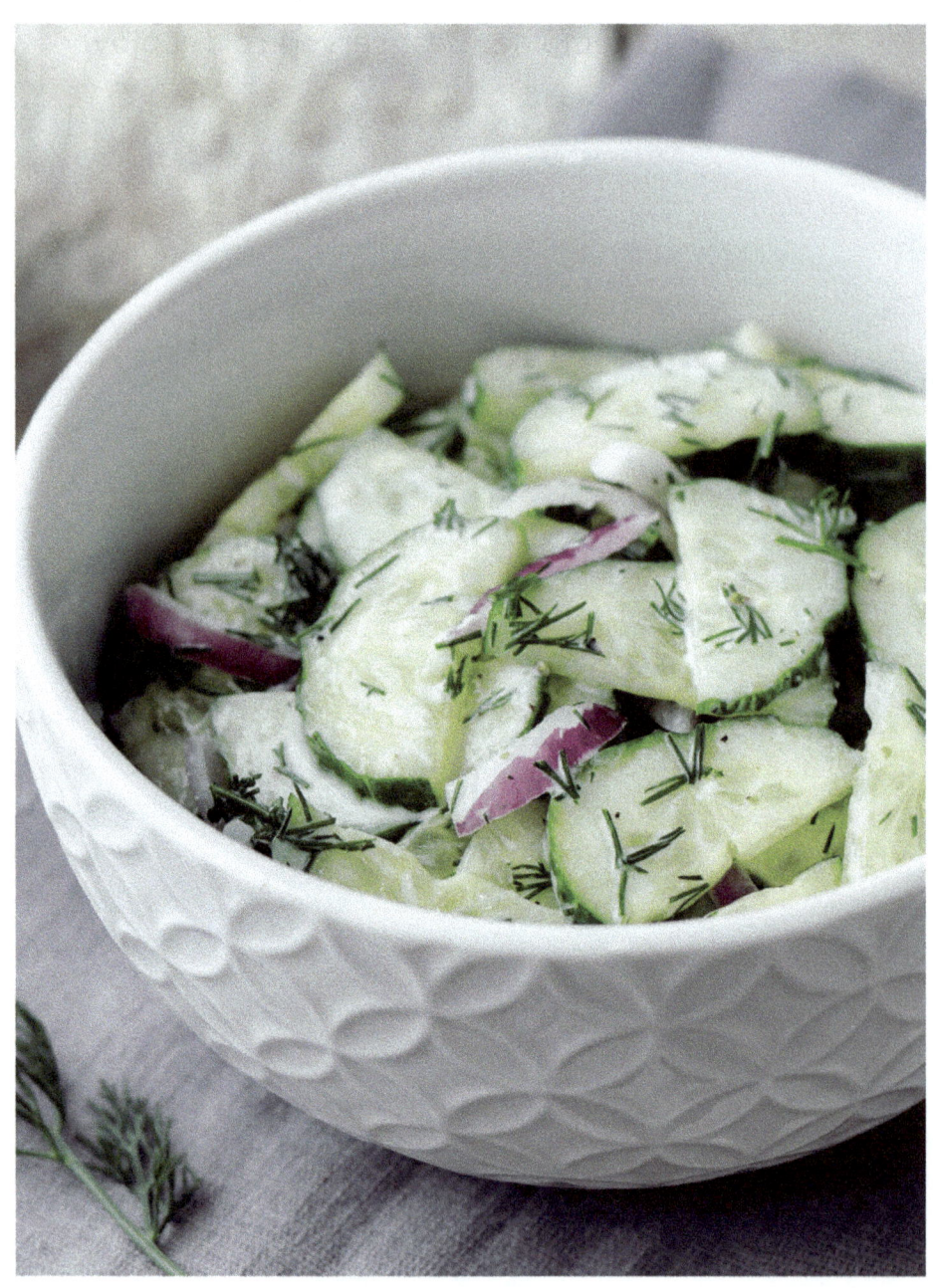

Carrot Salad with Yogurt

Servings: 4

Ingredients and Quantity

- 4 to 5 carrots, grated
- 3 garlic cloves, pressed
- 1/2 cup Greek yogurt
- 2 tbsp. mayonnaise
- 2 tbsp. olive oil
- 2 tbsp. finely chopped fresh dill
- Salt and pepper, to taste

Direction

1. Heat olive oil in a skillet and gently sauté carrots for 2 to 3 minutes or until wilted.

2. In a bowl, combine carrots, yogurt, mayonnaise, garlic and dill.

3. Add salt and black pepper to your taste.

4. Toss to combine. Serve and enjoy!

Strained Yogurt Salad

Servings: 4

Ingredients and Quantity

- 1 large or 2 small cucumbers, fresh or pickled
- 4 cups yogurt
- 2 to 3 crushed walnuts
- 1/2 bunch dill
- 3 tbsp. sunflower oil
- Salt, to taste

Direction

1. Strain the yogurt in a piece of cheesecloth or a clean white dishtowel.
2. You can suspend it over a bowl or the sink.

3. Peel and dice the cucumbers, place in a large bowl.
4. Add the crushed walnuts and the crushed garlic, the oil and the finely chopped dill.
5. Scoop the drained yogurt into the bowl and stir well.
6. Add salt to the taste, cover with cling film and put in the fridge for at least an hour so that the flavors can mix well. Serve and enjoy!

Turkish Beet Salad with Yogurt

Servings: 4

Ingredients and Quantity

- 3 medium beet roots
- 1 cup strained yogurt
- 1 garlic clove, minced
- 1 tsp. white vinegar or lemon juice
- 1 tbsp. extra virgin olive oil
- 1/4 tsp. dried mint
- 1/2 tsp. salt

Direction

1. Wash the beets well, cut the stems and steam in a pot or pan for 25 to 30 minutes or until properly cooked.

2. When they cool down, pat dry with paper towel.

3. Grate beets and put them in a deep bowl.

4. Add the other ingredients and toss. Best served cold. Enjoy!

Spinach Stem Salad

Servings: 2

Ingredients and Quantity

- Few bunches of spinach stems
- Water, for boiling the stems
- 1 garlic clove, minced
- Lemon juice or vinegar, to taste
- Extra virgin olive oil
- Salt, to taste

Direction

1. Trim the stems so that they will remain intact.
2. Wash the stems very well.

3. Steam the stems in a basket over boiling water for 2 to 3 minutes until wilted but not too fluffy.

4. Place them in a plate and sprinkle with minced garlic, olive oil, lemon juice or vinegar and salt. Serve and enjoy!

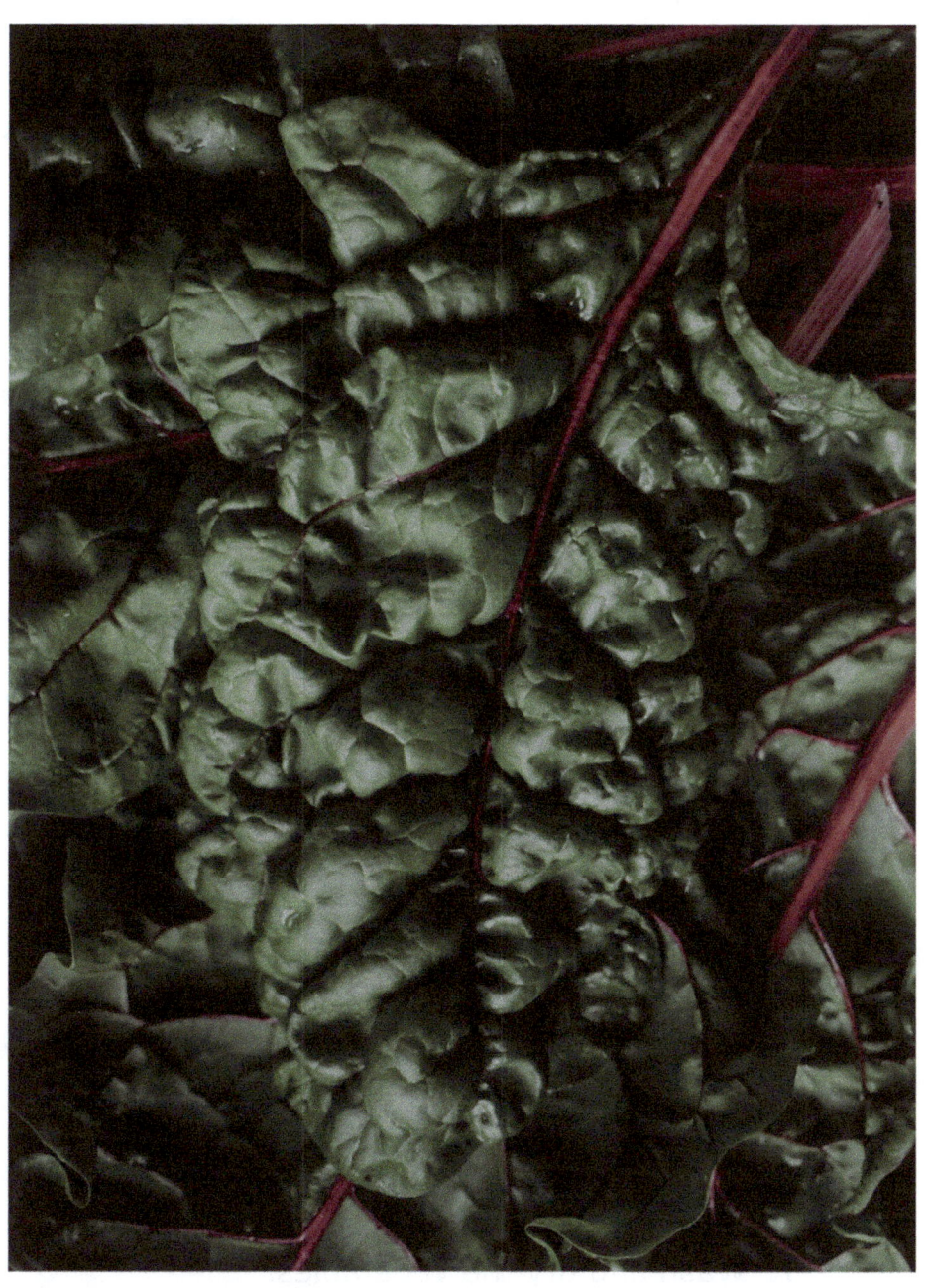

Roasted Eggplant and Pepper Relish

Servings: 4

Ingredients and Quantity

- 2 medium sized eggplants
- 2 red or green bell peppers
- 2 tomatoes
- 3 garlic cloves, crushed
- Some fresh parsley
- 1 to 2 tbsp. red wine vinegar
- Extra virgin oil, to taste
- Salt and pepper, to taste

Direction

1. Wash and dry the vegetables.
2. Prick the skin of the eggplants.

3. Bake the eggplants, tomatoes and peppers in a pre-heated oven at 400 F for about 40 minutes, until the skins are pretty burnt.
4. Take out of the oven and leave in a covered container for about 10 minutes.
5. Peel the skins off and drain well the extra juices.
6. De-seed the peppers.
7. Cut all the vegetables into small pieces.
8. Add the garlic and mix well with a fork or in a food processor.
9. Add the olive oil, vinegar and salt to taste. Stir again.
10. Serve cold and sprinkle parsley on top. Enjoy!

Kale Salad with Creamy Tahini Dressing

Servings: 4

Ingredients and Quantity

- 1 head kale
- 2 cucumbers, peeled and diced
- 1 avocado, peeled and diced
- 1 red onion, finely chopped
- 1 cup cherry tomatoes, halved

For the Dressing:

- 1/3 cup tahini
- /2 cup water
- garlic cloves, minced
- 3 tbsp. lemon juice
- 4 tbsp. extra virgin olive oil
- Salt and freshly ground black pepper, to taste

Direction

1. Prepare the dressing by whisking all ingredients.

2. Place all salad ingredients in a bowl and toss with the dressing.

3. Season to taste with black pepper and salt. Serve and enjoy!

Brown Lentil Salad

Servings: 4

Ingredients and Quantity

- 1 can lentils, drained and rinsed
- 1 red onion, thinly sliced
- 1 tomato, diced
- 1 red bell pepper, chopped
- 2 garlic cloves, crushed
- 2 tbsp. lemon juice
- 1/3 cup parsley leaves
- Salt and pepper, to taste

Direction

1. Place lentils, red onion, tomatoes, bell pepper and lemon juice in a large bowl.
2. Season with salt and black pepper to taste.

3. Toss to combine and sprinkle with parsley.

   Serve and enjoy!

Bulgur with Walnuts and Green Lentils

Servings: 4

Ingredients and Quantity

- 1 cup bulgur
- 1 cup hot water
- 1/2 cup cooked green lentils
- 1/2 cup walnuts, crushed
- 1 cup halved cherry tomatoes
- 1 red or green, pepper, cut
- 3 to 4 spring onion, finely cut
- /2 cup parsley, finely cut
- 1 tbsp. dried mint
- 1 tsp. dried basil
- 3 tbsp. extra virgin olive oil
- Salt and pepper, to taste

Direction

1. In a bowl, combine bulgur, hot water and olive oil.
2. Stir, cover and set aside for 15 minutes to steam.
3. Add in lentils, walnuts, onions, pepper, tomatoes and salt to your taste.
4. Also add the parsley, dried basil and mint.
5. Toss to combine. Serve and enjoy!

Slimming Ginger Steamed Fish

Preparation time: 20 Minutes

Ingredients

- 1/2 red pepper julienned
- 1 large clove garlic sliced thinly
- 1 tablespoon soy sauce
- 1/2 tablespoon mirin
- 1 tablespoon sesame oil
- 1/2 tsp. Thai chili deseeded and sliced very thin
- 2 5oz fillets halibut or other white fish
- 1 tsp. Salt
- 3 scallions julienned
- 2 tablespoon ginger julienned

Directions

1. Place one of the fillets in a heatproof bowl that will fit in your steamer, and top with half of the salt, scallions, ginger, red peppers and garlic.
2. Place another fillet on top of the first and repeat the process with the remaining ingredients.
3. Add the chili, soy sauce, and mirin and sesame oil.
4. Put 1 inch of water in the bottom a pot over medium heat and place steamer in the pot.
5. Place the bowl with the fish in the steamer (the water should not be touching the steamer or the bowl) and cover the pot.
6. Steam the fish for 15-20 minutes depending on the thickness of your fillets.
7. Serve with brown rice and half a lemon.

One Pan Baked Teriyaki Salmon

Preparation time: 30 Minutes

Ingredients

- 1/2 lb. salmon fillet
- 2 zucchini cut into small cubes
- 2 carrots cut into 2 small cubes
- 1 tablespoon salt course
- 1 1/2 tablespoon sesame oil
- 2 tablespoon scallions chopped (green parts only)
- 1 tablespoon sesame seeds
- 1 tablespoon ginger peeled and cut into matchsticks
- 2 cloves garlic
- 1/2 tablespoon corn starch
- 2/3 cup pineapple cubed
- 1/2 orange sliced into 6 slices
- 1/2 cup soy sauce
- 1/4 cup mirin

- 2 tablespoon maple syrup
- 1/2 orange juiced

Directions

1. Pre-heat oven to 400°F.
2. In a pot over medium heat, combine the soy sauce, mirin, orange juice and bring to a boil. Reduce heat and add the pineapple and stir until thick.
3. Lay the salmon fillet skin side down on a baking sheet covered in parchment paper and slide the orange under the fillet halfway. Surround the outside of the fillet with the zucchini and carrot.
4. Season with salt and the sesame oil and pour the marinade on top of the salmon fillet saving a little to dress the dish at the end.
5. Bake for 15 minutes then broil for 5 minutes or until the top is caramelized, then garnish with

more sauce, scallions and sesame seeds. Serve and enjoy!

Blackened Fish Tacos with Cabbage Mango Slaw

Preparation time: 45 Minutes

Ingredients

For Tacos:

- 1 lb. skinless cod or halibut filet
- 1/2 lime, juiced
- Cooking spray
- 8 corn tortillas
- Lime wedges for serving
- 1/2 lime, cut into wedges
- 1/4 tsp. (1/2 tsp. for spicier) ground cayenne pepper
- 1/4 tsp. ground cumin
- 1/4 tsp. ground oregano
- 1/8 tsp. black pepper
- 1 tsp. smoked paprika

- 1 tsp. kosher salt
- ½ tsp. dry mustard

For Cabbage Slaw:

- 3 1/2 cups (1/2 small) red cabbage, shredded fine
- 1 mango, julienned
- 2 tsp. olive oil
- 1/4 cup cilantro
- 1/2 tsp. kosher salt
- 1 lime, juiced

Directions

1. Combine all the slaw ingredients and refrigerate.
2. In a small bowl, mix the dried spices and seasoning together, squeeze the lime on the fish then rub the seasoning onto fish.
3. On grill or stove on high heat, heat a cast iron skillet till really hot. Spray with nonstick oil spray.

4. Cook fish for about 5mins on each side until opaque in the center and well browned on the outside. Heat the corn tortillas on the grill for about 1 to 2 minutes or until they slightly char.
5. Cut the fish into 8 pieces (or you can flake it if it's easier).
6. Divide the fish equally between 8 tortillas and top each with 1/2 cup slaw. Serve with lime wedges.

Garlic Lemon Scallops

Preparation time: 30 Minutes

Ingredients

- 1 pinch ground sage
- 1 lemon, juiced
- 2 tbsp. parsley, chopped
- 1 lb. scallops
- 2 tbsps. All-purpose flour
- 1 tbsp. olive oil
- 4 garlic cloves, minced
- 1 scallion, finely chopped

Directions

1. Heat the oil in a large non- stick skillet.
2. Toss scallops with flour and salt, in a medium bowl

3. Place scallops in the skillet; add garlic, scallions, and sage.

4. Sauté for about 3-4hrs or until scallops are just opaque

5. Stir in lemon juice and parsley; remove from heat and serve immediately.

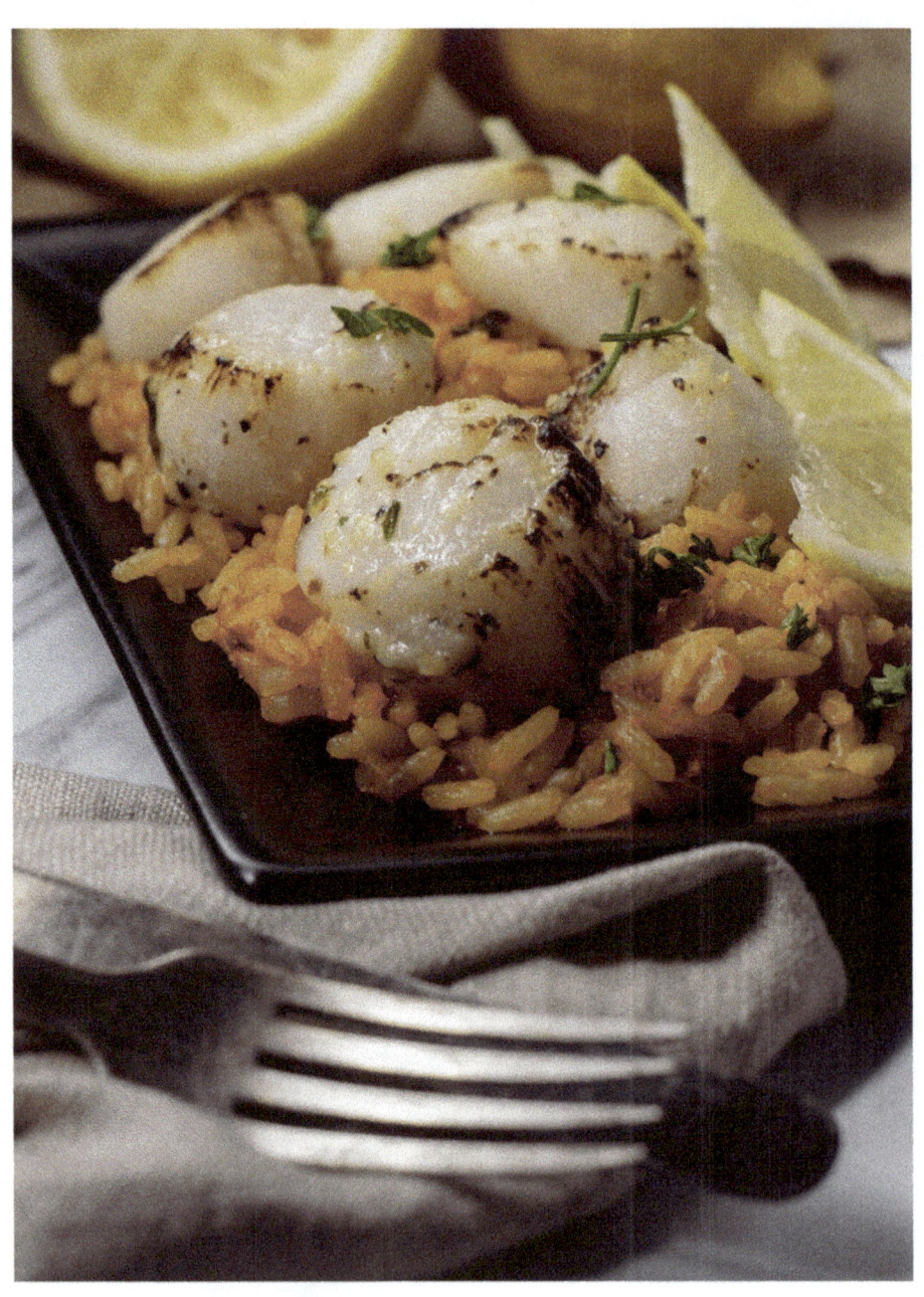

Shrimp & Broccoli in Chili Sauce

Preparation: 95 Minutes

Ingredients

- 2 teaspoon corn starch
- 2 teaspoon sugar
- 1/2 teaspoon salt
- 1 tablespoon oil
- 3 cup broccoli, cut into florets
- 4 cup cooked soba noodles,
- 8 oz. uncooked buckwheat noodles, or vermicelli
- 2 tablespoons dry sherry
- 1 1/2 teaspoons paprika
- 1/2 teaspoon ground red pepper
- 4 garlic cloves, crushed
- 1/3 cup water
- 1/4 cup chili sauce (like Heinz)
- 2 lb. medium shrimp, peeled and deveined

- 2 tablespoons minced seeded jalapeño pepper (about 2 peppers)

Directions

1. In a medium bowl, combine shrimp, jalapeno pepper, sherry, paprika, red pepper and garlic cloves and chill for 1 hour
2. Combine water, chili sauce, corn starch, sugar, salt and oil in another bowl and set aside.
3. Heat oil in a stir fry pan. Add Broccoli and stir fry for 2mins.
4. Add shrimp mixture, stir fry 5 minutes or until shrimp are done, then add cornstarch mixture and bring to a boil. Cook for 1 minute or until sauce thickens.
5. Serve over soba noodles.

Prawn Pitta Scoops

Preparation time: 10 Minutes

Ingredients

- Juice of ½ lemon
- 2 tablespoon fresh coriander leaves
- 160 g (5½ oz.) cooked, peeled prawns
- ½ tsp. paprika
- Salt and freshly ground black pepper to season
- 125g (4¼ oz.) avocado, peeled, stoned and finely chopped
- 200g (7 oz.) tomatoes, quartered, deseeded and finely chopped
- ½ small red onion, finely chopped
- 4 pitta breads

Directions

1. Preheat the grill to high.
2. Meanwhile, open out the Pitta Breads and slice each half in 2 to make 16 pitta scoops.
3. Place on a grill pan, and grill for 4-5 minutes or until golden and toasted.
4. Combine the chopped avocado, tomatoes, onion, lemon juice and coriander and season.
5. Divide the avocado mix between the pitta scoops. Top with the prawns and a pinch of paprika.
6. Serve!

Shrimp with Cilantro and Lime

Preparation time: 40 Minutes

Ingredients

- 1 1/2 pounds peeled and deveined jumbo shrimp
- 2 tablespoons lime juice (from 1 medium lime)
- 2 garlic cloves, crushed
- 3 to 4 tablespoons chopped fresh cilantro
- 1 tablespoon olive oil
- 1 teaspoon lime, zest
- Salt and pepper, to taste

Directions

1. In a large bowl, combine shrimp, lime juice, cumin, ginger, and garlic. Toss well.

3. Heat oil in a large nonstick skillet over medium-high heat.

4. Add shrimp mixture and sauté until shrimp is done, about 4mins

5. Remove from heat and stir in cilantro, lime zest, salt, and pepper.

6. Serve!

Maple Mustard Salmon

Servings: 4

Ingredients

- 2 tbsp. maple syrup (pure)
- Salt and pepper
- 1.33 lb. raw wild salmon
- 3 tbsp. whole grain mustard

Directions

1. Preheat the oven to 350 degrees F.
2. Mix together the maple syrup and mustard.
3. Brush over the salmon. Bake for 10-12 minutes until cooked to your liking.

Grilled Shrimp Marinade with Shrimp Sauce

Servings: 5

Ingredients

- ½ teaspoon salt
- ½ teaspoon pepper
- Pinch of red pepper flakes

For Sauce:

- 1 tablespoon prepared horseradish sauce
- 2 tablespoons ketchup
- 1 tablespoon non-fat plain Greek yogurt
- 24 medium Shrimp cleaned and deveined
- 2 teaspoons balsamic vinegar
- 1 teaspoon olive oil
- Juice of 1 lemon
- 1 clove garlic minced

Directions

1. In a medium bowl, mix together vinegar, oil, lemon juice, garlic, salt, pepper, and pepper flakes in a medium bowl.
2. Pour over shrimp then covers and refrigerate for a minimum of half an hour.
3. Slide shrimp onto skewers.
4. Grill for 2-3 minutes on each side. Shrimp cooks fast, so watch for it to curl and turn pink.

For Sauce:

1. In a small bowl, mix together all ingredients.
2. Add more or less horseradish sauce to taste

Mexi' Shrimp Salad Wrap

Servings: 4

Ingredients

- 1/2 cup finely chopped romaine lettuce
- 3 tbsp. fresh salsa or pico de gallo
- 2 tbsp. canned black beans, drained and rinsed
- 2 tbsp. frozen corn kernels, thawed
- 2 tbsp. chopped fresh cilantro
- 1 medium-large high-fiber flour tortilla with 110 calories or less
- 2 tbsp. fat-free sour cream
- 1/2 tbsp. fresh lime juice
- 1/8 tsp. ground cumin
- 2 dashes chili powder, or more to taste
- 3 oz. cooked and chopped shrimp

Directions

1. Mix sour cream, lime juice, cumin, chili powder and, if you like, a dash of salt in a large bowl. Stir in all remaining ingredients except tortilla.
2. Spoon mixture across the center of the tortilla.
3. Wrap tortilla up by first folding one side in (to keep filling from escaping), and then tightly rolling it up from the bottom. Enjoy!

Fish and Shrimp Stew

Servings: 4

Ingredients

- 8 oz. clam juice
- 14 oz. fish stock
- 2 tbsp. almond butter (or ghee for Whole 30)
- 1/2 tsp. oregano
- 1/2 tsp. Basil
- Salt and pepper
- 1 tbsp. olive oil
- 1 onion, diced
- 2 garlic cloves, minced
- 1/4 tsp. red pepper flakes (optional, I used double, that's for a spicier soup)
- 2/3 cup parsley
- 3 tbsp. tomato paste
- 28 oz. canned San Marzano tomatoes

Directions

1. Heat the olive oil over medium heat. Add the onion and cook for 5-7 minutes until beginning to become translucent.
2. Add the garlic and red pepper flakes. Cook for 1-2 minutes, stirring often. Add the parsley and cook for 1-2 minutes. Stir in the tomato paste and cook for 1 minute.
3. Add the tomatoes, clam juice, and fish stock. Bring to a simmer and add the butter, oregano, and basil. Simmer for 10-15 minutes. At this point, you want to taste the broth and adjust the seasoning as needed.
4. Add salt and pepper. If needed, add extra tomato paste for more tomato flavor. You can add red pepper flakes for more heat or some extra tomatoes if it is too spicy.

5. Make sure the broth is simmering and add the cod. Cook for 5 minutes. Then add the shrimp and cook for 4-5 minutes until opaque and cooked through.

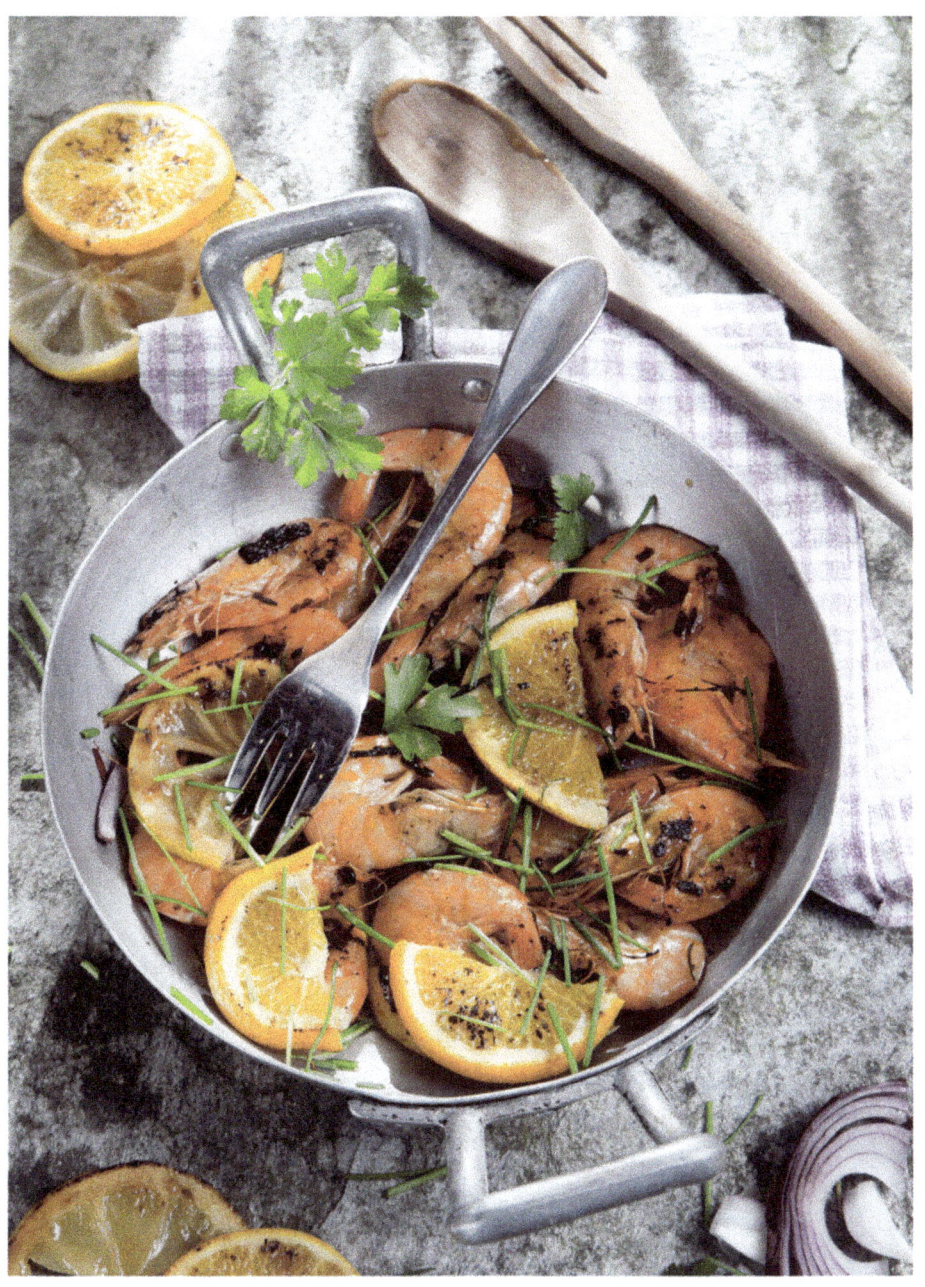

www.ingramcontent.com/pod-product-compliance
Lightning Source LLC
Chambersburg PA
CBHW070733030426
42336CB00013B/1964